I0477376

UNDERSTANDING

TRANSCRANIAL

MAGNETIC

STIMULATION

FOR BEGINNERS

From Principles To Practice:
Unlocking The Power Of Non-
Invasive Brain Therapy For Mental
Health, Depression, Anxiety, And
Beyond

DR. ALICIA SONYA

CONTENTS

Copyright © 2024, By Dr. Alicia Sonya

All Rights Reserved.

No part of this book may be reproduced, stored in a retrieval system, or transmitted in any form or by any means—electronic, mechanical, photocopying, recording, or otherwise—without prior written permission from the publisher, except in the case of brief quotations embodied in critical reviews and certain other noncommercial uses permitted by copyright law.

DISCLAIMER

The information provided in this book is for educational and informational purposes only and is not intended as medical advice, diagnosis, or treatment. Always consult with a qualified healthcare professional before beginning any therapy, practice, or lifestyle change.

The author and publisher of this book make no representations or warranties regarding the accuracy, applicability, or completeness of the content presented. While every effort has been made to ensure the information provided is accurate and up-to-date, the field of health and wellness is constantly evolving, and the reader is advised to use discretion and seek professional guidance as needed.

This book contains references to individuals, products, websites, organizations, or other entities solely for informational purposes. The author and publisher do not endorse, sponsor, or affiliate with any of these references, nor do they receive any benefit from their inclusion. The mention of any names, trademarks, or products does not imply any association or endorsement.

The use of this book is solely at the reader's discretion. Neither the author nor the publisher shall be held liable for any damages, loss, or injury resulting from the use or misuse of the information contained herein.

ABOUT THIS BOOK

Understanding Transcranial Magnetic Stimulation For Beginners" serves as an essential resource for anyone seeking a thorough understanding of this innovative brain stimulation therapy. Transcranial Magnetic Stimulation (TMS) has garnered significant attention due to its non-invasive nature and its growing applications in treating various mental health conditions.

Beginning with an introduction to TMS, this book offers readers a foundational overview of what TMS is and how it works. By comparing it to other brain stimulation techniques, readers can grasp the unique mechanisms and advantages of TMS, alongside a historical perspective on its evolution in mental health treatment. This background sets the stage for a deeper exploration of who can benefit from TMS, offering clear insights into the range of individuals and conditions that may find relief through this therapy.

In the exploration of how TMS works, this book dives into the mechanics of magnetic fields and their role in stimulating neurons. Readers will gain a detailed understanding of how TMS affects brain function and the different types of TMS available, including rTMS, iTMS, and dTMS. Each method is explained about how they target specific brain regions, enabling readers to comprehend the tailored nature of TMS treatments.

Additionally, this book highlights the long-term effects of TMS on brain activity, giving readers a sense of the lasting impact it can have on neurological function.

A significant portion of the book is dedicated to the clinical applications of TMS. With an emphasis on depression, anxiety, PTSD, and OCD, this guide provides a comprehensive look at the clinical evidence supporting TMS's effectiveness in these areas.

Emerging uses for TMS in treating conditions such as bipolar disorder, ADHD, chronic pain, and migraines are also covered, showcasing the expanding scope of this technology. Readers will appreciate the clear explanations of how TMS is adapted to meet the needs of various conditions, backed by the latest research and clinical findings.

For those considering TMS, this book provides a detailed guide to the treatment process, including what to expect during consultations and preparation for sessions. The step-by-step breakdown of the treatment itself, session length, and overall treatment duration equips readers with practical knowledge, reducing any anxiety about the unknown. Moreover, this guide covers frequency and duration recommendations, helping individuals understand what their treatment plans might look like.

When it comes to equipment, this book offers an insightful overview of TMS machines and their components, from coils to control systems. Readers will learn about the safety features integrated into modern TMS equipment, ensuring a safe treatment experience. Innovations in TMS technology are also explored, including the development of home-based TMS devices and whether they are safe for use outside clinical settings.

The effectiveness of TMS is a critical topic, and this book offers a well-rounded discussion of the benefits associated with this treatment. Comparing TMS with traditional medications and psychotherapy allows readers to see where TMS stands in the spectrum of mental health interventions. This guide also highlights success rates, patient experiences, and how quickly individuals might see results, offering reassurance to those curious about its efficacy.

Additionally, it provides strategies for maintaining mental health after completing a course of TMS.

Concerns about side effects are thoroughly addressed, including the discomfort some individuals may experience during treatment and potential side effects such as headaches. This book also advises on how to manage these minor side effects while detailing who should avoid TMS due to contraindications. For those concerned about cognitive impacts, the guide provides clear information on whether TMS can affect memory or cause brain damage, addressing common fears with factual reassurance.

Cost, insurance, and accessibility are vital considerations for anyone contemplating TMS.

This book breaks down the financial aspects of TMS treatment, from the cost of sessions to the specifics of insurance coverage, including Medicare and Medicaid options. Readers will also find practical advice on locating TMS clinics, as well as information on financial assistance and payment plans that can make this life-changing treatment more accessible.

This guide answers frequently asked questions in a clear, accessible manner, helping individuals assess whether they are good candidates for TMS, how it feels during treatment, and whether they can combine TMS with medications. It also covers the possibility of needing maintenance TMS and whether there's any downtime after sessions, ensuring that readers are fully informed about the day-to-day realities of undergoing TMS.

Looking ahead, this book explores future trends and innovations in TMS, including research into new applications for the technology and the growing potential of personalized TMS treatments.

The role of artificial intelligence and data in improving outcomes is also discussed, highlighting how technological advancements are enhancing the effectiveness and accessibility of TMS. With a focus on lowering costs and expanding the reach of TMS to more individuals, this book positions TMS as a forward-thinking solution in the evolving field of mental health care.

CHAPTER ONE

Introduction To Transcranial Magnetic Stimulation (TMS)

Transcranial Magnetic Stimulation (TMS) is a non-invasive brain stimulation technique that uses magnetic fields to stimulate nerve cells in the brain. It is commonly used to treat depression, especially in individuals who have not responded well to traditional treatments like medications or therapy. The process involves placing a magnetic coil near the scalp, usually over the prefrontal cortex, which generates pulses that penetrate the skull and target specific areas of the brain.

The procedure is done while the patient is awake, and seated in a comfortable chair, and it typically lasts about 30 to 60 minutes per session. There is no need for anesthesia or sedation. TMS is considered a safe and effective alternative to more invasive treatments such as electroconvulsive therapy (ECT) and is associated with fewer side effects. Patients often require multiple sessions over the course of several weeks to achieve noticeable improvements in their symptoms.

Common side effects are mild and may include headaches, scalp discomfort, or tingling sensations at the stimulation site. These usually resolve shortly after the session. Because TMS is non-invasive and has minimal downtime, patients can resume their normal activities immediately after the procedure.

Overview Of TMS: What Is It?

Transcranial Magnetic Stimulation (TMS) is a medical procedure used to treat neurological and psychiatric conditions by stimulating brain regions using magnetic pulses. The device generates a magnetic field that creates small electric currents in the brain, altering the activity of neurons. This technique is primarily used for treating major depressive disorder (MDD) but has applications in conditions like anxiety, OCD, and even chronic pain.

TMS involves positioning an electromagnetic coil on the patient's head, targeting a specific brain region—usually the dorsolateral prefrontal cortex, which plays a key role in mood regulation. The magnetic pulses penetrate the skull, activating nerve cells in that area. Each session typically lasts between 20 to 40 minutes, and treatments are repeated daily over four to six weeks to achieve results.

Unlike medications that affect the entire brain chemically, TMS focuses on a localized area, which reduces the risk of systemic side effects. Most patients experience only mild discomfort during the procedure, and it does not require hospitalization or anesthesia, making it a convenient outpatient treatment.

The Science Behind TMS: How It Works
TMS works by using electromagnetic fields to influence the electrical activity in specific parts of the brain. The magnetic pulses are delivered through a coil placed on the scalp. When the coil emits these pulses, they create an electric current that stimulates neurons in

the targeted brain area. This can increase or decrease the activity of these neurons, depending on the frequency and intensity of the magnetic pulses.

The most commonly targeted area is the dorsolateral prefrontal cortex, which is involved in mood regulation. For people with depression, this region often shows reduced activity. TMS aims to "reset" the electrical activity, increasing neuronal firing and improving mood regulation. Over time, repeated stimulation helps normalize brain activity, leading to improved mental health outcomes.

Research shows that TMS can induce lasting changes in brain connectivity, enhancing synaptic plasticity and neural networks involved in emotional and cognitive processing. This makes TMS particularly effective for treatment-resistant depression, where other therapies have failed.

TMS Vs. Other Brain Stimulation Techniques

TMS differs from other brain stimulation methods, such as Electroconvulsive Therapy (ECT) and Deep Brain Stimulation (DBS), in both its approach and invasiveness. While ECT uses electrical currents to cause a seizure, TMS uses magnetic fields to modulate brain activity without causing seizures. This makes TMS a less risky and more comfortable option for many patients, as it doesn't require anesthesia or result in memory loss, which is a common side effect of ECT.

Deep Brain Stimulation (DBS), on the other hand, involves surgically implanting electrodes in the brain, which deliver electrical impulses to regulate brain activity. This procedure is more invasive and typically used for severe cases of Parkinson's disease or epilepsy. In contrast, TMS is non-invasive, allowing for easier and more accessible outpatient treatments.

In terms of effectiveness, while ECT is considered more effective for severe depression, TMS offers a balance between efficacy and tolerability, making it a preferred option for patients seeking non-invasive alternatives. Furthermore, TMS has fewer cognitive side effects and a shorter recovery time compared to other stimulation techniques.

History And Evolution Of TMS In Mental Health

TMS was first introduced in 1985 by Anthony Barker and his colleagues, who developed it as a tool for brain mapping and studying the motor cortex. In its early stages, TMS was used primarily for research purposes, exploring how different areas of the brain responded to stimulation. By the late 1990s, researchers began to explore its potential therapeutic applications, particularly in treating mental health disorders like depression.

In 2008, the U.S. Food and Drug Administration (FDA) approved TMS as a treatment for depression, marking a turning point for its use in clinical practice. Since then, TMS has evolved with improved technology and protocols, expanding its applications beyond depression to include conditions like obsessive-compulsive disorder (OCD), post-traumatic stress disorder (PTSD), and chronic pain.

Over the years, TMS has gained widespread acceptance due to its non-invasive nature and positive outcomes for treatment-resistant conditions.

Today, ongoing research is exploring its use in other areas, including schizophrenia, bipolar disorder, and cognitive enhancement, further solidifying its role in modern mental health care.

Who Can Benefit From TMS?

TMS is primarily used for patients who have not found relief from traditional treatments like antidepressant medications or psychotherapy. It is especially beneficial for individuals with treatment-resistant depression, offering an alternative when other therapies have failed. TMS is also being used to treat other mental health disorders like obsessive-compulsive disorder (OCD) and anxiety.

People who are unable to tolerate the side effects of medications, such as weight gain, sexual dysfunction, or fatigue, may also find TMS to be a suitable option. The treatment is well-tolerated, with fewer side effects compared to medications, and does not affect the whole body since it targets a specific brain region.

However, not everyone is eligible for TMS. Individuals with metal implants in or near the head, a history of seizures, or certain neurological conditions may not be suitable candidates. A thorough evaluation by a healthcare provider is necessary to determine if TMS is an appropriate and safe option for a particular individual.

CHAPTER TWO

Understanding The Mechanism Of TMS

Transcranial Magnetic Stimulation (TMS) uses magnetic fields to stimulate nerve cells in the brain. During the procedure, a coil is placed near the scalp, generating magnetic pulses that pass through the skull to target specific areas of the brain. These pulses create electric currents, which activate neurons without causing pain or lasting damage to the brain tissue.

The procedure is typically non-invasive and doesn't require anesthesia. It can be performed in an outpatient setting, with patients remaining awake and seated throughout the session.

Sessions usually last around 30 to 40 minutes, and patients may undergo multiple sessions over several weeks to achieve the desired therapeutic effects.

TMS is primarily used to treat conditions like depression, anxiety, and neurological disorders. The stimulation helps in modulating the activity of brain regions that may be underactive or overactive, restoring balance and improving symptoms. It's a safe procedure with minimal side effects, typically limited to mild discomfort or a headache.

Magnetic Fields And Neuronal Stimulation

TMS relies on magnetic fields to generate electrical impulses in the brain. These magnetic pulses are created by a coil placed near the scalp, which rapidly alternates magnetic fields. This change induces electric currents in the brain's neurons, prompting them to fire.

This electrical activity causes neurons to depolarize, affecting their communication with surrounding neurons. The stimulation can either increase or decrease neuronal activity depending on the frequency and intensity of the magnetic pulses. High-frequency stimulation often increases activity, while low-frequency stimulation tends to reduce it.

The key advantage of TMS is its precision. The magnetic fields can be directed at very specific brain areas, minimizing effects on non-target regions. This allows for a focused treatment of conditions like depression, where stimulating particular areas of the prefrontal cortex can help regulate mood.

How TMS Affects Brain Function

TMS affects brain function by modulating the activity of neurons in targeted regions. For example, in treating depression, TMS is often applied to the left dorsolateral prefrontal cortex, an area associated with mood regulation. By stimulating this area, TMS increases neural activity, potentially reversing the interactivity that's often seen in depressed patients.

Repeated TMS sessions can lead to lasting changes in brain connectivity and plasticity. These changes help "rewire" the brain, promoting healthier patterns of neuronal communication.

Over time, this can result in improvements in mood, cognitive function, or motor control, depending on the condition being treated.

Additionally, TMS can affect neurotransmitter release, increasing levels of chemicals like dopamine and serotonin. These neurotransmitters play a key role in mood and motivation, which is why TMS is considered effective for mental health conditions such as major depressive disorder and anxiety.

Types Of TMS: RTMS, ITMS, DTMS Explained.

Repetitive TMS (rTMS) involves delivering pulses in rapid succession at regular intervals. This is the most common form used for treating depression and is designed to repeatedly stimulate the same brain region to promote long-lasting changes in brain activity. rTMS sessions are typically scheduled over a series of weeks, with patients receiving daily treatments.

Intermittent TMS (iTMS) works similarly to rTMS but involves periods of rest between pulses, allowing the brain to "reset" between stimulations. This variation is often used in research settings to explore how different frequencies and patterns of stimulation can affect brain function. It can be more comfortable for patients who are sensitive to continuous stimulation.

Deep TMS (dTMS) uses a specialized coil to penetrate deeper brain regions that are typically out of reach with standard TMS. It's often used to target areas involved in more complex brain functions, like decision-making and emotion regulation. TMS is becoming more popular as an option for patients who do not respond to traditional rTMS, offering a broader range of therapeutic possibilities.

Targeting Different Brain Areas With TMS

The area of the brain targeted during TMS depends on the condition being treated. For depression, the dorsolateral prefrontal cortex (DLPFC) is often stimulated, as it is involved in regulating mood. For motor disorders like Parkinson's, the motor cortex may be the focus, aiming to improve movement and coordination by stimulating the areas responsible for controlling muscles.

When planning treatment, a clinician will use MRI or other brain mapping techniques to identify the most relevant brain region for stimulation. This ensures that the TMS pulses are directed with precision to the specific area that needs modulation. The process may involve some trial and error, especially when treating conditions like anxiety, where different regions of the brain might be involved.

The ability to target different brain areas also makes TMS useful for a wide variety of neurological and psychiatric conditions. By fine-tuning the location and intensity of the stimulation, TMS can be adapted to treat disorders ranging from PTSD to chronic pain syndromes.

Long-Term Effects Of TMS On Brain Activity

TMS can lead to long-term changes in brain activity, especially with repeated sessions. The process of repeated stimulation promotes neuroplasticity, the brain's ability to reorganize itself by forming new neural connections. This is particularly important for treating conditions like depression, where certain brain circuits may be underactive.

Patients often experience a cumulative effect, with symptoms continuing to improve even after the TMS treatment course has ended. In many cases, the benefits can last for months, although booster sessions may be necessary to maintain these effects over time. This prolonged benefit is due to the sustained changes in brain chemistry and neuron communication   initiated   by   repeated stimulation.

While TMS is generally considered safe, its long-term effects on brain health are still being studied. Current research suggests that TMS does not cause lasting negative effects on brain function, and it may even promote brain health by enhancing plasticity and improving connectivity between different brain regions.

CHAPTER THREE

Conditions Treated By TMS

Transcranial Magnetic Stimulation (TMS) is commonly used to treat various mental health conditions, especially when traditional treatments like medication and therapy have not been effective.

The most well-known application is for major depressive disorder (MDD), where it is used to stimulate parts of the brain that are underactive. Beyond depression, TMS has been used to treat conditions like anxiety, obsessive-compulsive disorder (OCD), and post-traumatic stress disorder (PTSD).

For each condition, the specific area of the brain targeted by TMS differs slightly. For instance, in depression, the left prefrontal cortex is typically stimulated because this region is often less active in people with depression.

In anxiety disorders, the focus shifts to different regions of the brain involved in emotional regulation. While treatment protocols vary by condition, the overall goal is to restore balanced brain activity.

In clinical practice, TMS is also being explored for a wide range of emerging uses, including chronic pain syndromes, bipolar disorder, and even migraines. This makes TMS a versatile tool in modern psychiatric and neurological care, offering new hope for patients with conditions that have proven resistant to other therapies.

TMS For Depression: Clinical Evidence

TMS has shown strong clinical evidence in the treatment of depression, especially for individuals who have not responded to antidepressants. Studies indicate that TMS is effective in about 50-60% of cases, with many patients experiencing significant improvement after a course of treatment. This makes TMS an attractive option for those seeking an alternative to medication-based interventions.

The treatment involves delivering magnetic pulses to the left prefrontal cortex, a region of the brain that controls mood regulation. These pulses help stimulate neural activity in areas that are underactive in people with depression. Sessions typically last 30 to 40 minutes, and patients usually undergo treatment five times a week for four to six weeks. The gradual build-up of stimulation over these sessions helps to restore healthy brain function.

Side effects of TMS are generally mild and include headaches or scalp discomfort, which usually resolves after treatment. Unlike medications, TMS does not cause systemic side effects like weight gain or sexual dysfunction, making it a preferred option for some patients.

The non-invasive nature of TMS has made it a breakthrough therapy in treating depression, offering real results without the need for surgery or medication.

Anxiety And Panic Disorders: TMS Applications

TMS is also increasingly being used to treat anxiety and panic disorders, targeting the brain areas involved in fear and stress responses. For anxiety, the right prefrontal cortex is often the focus because this area tends to be overactive in individuals with anxiety. By delivering targeted magnetic pulses, TMS helps to balance this brain activity and reduce anxiety symptoms.

The procedure for treating anxiety with TMS is similar to that for depression. Patients undergo daily sessions over the course of several weeks, with each session lasting around 30 minutes. The treatment is painless, and patients can resume normal activities immediately afterward.

Many people report feeling calmer and less anxious after several sessions, as the brain gradually adjusts to the repeated stimulation.

Clinical studies are ongoing, but early results show promise for treating not only generalized anxiety disorder but also panic disorder. This non-invasive treatment is particularly valuable for patients who have not responded well to medications, offering a drug-free alternative with minimal side effects.

TMS For PTSD And OCD

TMS has been explored as a treatment option for PTSD (post-traumatic stress disorder) and OCD (obsessive-compulsive disorder), two conditions that often resist standard therapies. In PTSD, the brain's overactivity in response to trauma is targeted, particularly in the amygdala and prefrontal cortex, which are involved in fear and stress responses. By using TMS, clinicians aim to reduce the heightened reactions these brain areas have to traumatic memories.

For OCD, the focus is on reducing activity in the brain's cortico-striatal circuit, which is hyperactive in individuals with obsessive thoughts and compulsive behaviors. Patients typically receive TMS targeting the supplementary motor area, a region associated with these behaviors.

TMS is conducted daily over several weeks, and while results may take time, many patients experience significant reductions in their OCD symptoms.

Both conditions have shown promising responses to TMS in clinical trials. Although not a first-line treatment, TMS offers hope for patients with PTSD and OCD, especially those who have found medications and traditional therapy ineffective.

Emerging Uses: Bipolar Disorder, ADHD, And More

TMS is increasingly being studied for conditions beyond depression and anxiety, including bipolar disorder and attention-deficit/hyperactivity disorder (ADHD). In bipolar disorder, TMS is used to manage depressive episodes, though care is taken to avoid triggering manic phases. The precise brain regions targeted in bipolar disorder treatment vary depending on the patient's symptoms and mood cycle.

For ADHD, TMS is thought to improve attention and impulse control by stimulating underactive areas of the brain, particularly the dorsolateral prefrontal cortex. Though research is still in the early stages, initial studies suggest that TMS may improve focus and cognitive function in people with ADHD, offering an alternative to medication.

Emerging research is also exploring TMS for a variety of other conditions, including autism spectrum disorder, schizophrenia, and even substance use disorders.

While much of this work is still experimental, the potential for TMS to address a broad range of psychiatric and neurological issues is exciting, offering new avenues for treatment in the future.

Can TMS Help With Chronic Pain And Migraines?

TMS has shown promise in treating chronic pain and migraines, conditions that affect millions of people worldwide. For chronic pain, TMS works by targeting the motor cortex, the area of the brain that controls movement, which is believed to influence the perception of pain. Regular TMS sessions can help modulate the brain's response to pain signals, providing relief for conditions like fibromyalgia and neuropathic pain.

When used for migraines, TMS is applied to the occipital cortex, the area of the brain responsible for visual processing, which is often implicated in migraine headaches. Patients typically use TMS as a preventive treatment, undergoing sessions a few times a week to reduce the frequency and intensity of migraines. Portable TMS devices have also been developed for home use, allowing patients to treat themselves at the onset of a migraine.

While TMS may not eliminate pain or migraines, it can significantly improve the quality of life for sufferers who have not responded to other treatments. With ongoing research, TMS continues to offer new hope for people living with chronic pain and debilitating migraines.

CHAPTER FOUR

The TMS Procedure: What To Expect

Transcranial Magnetic Stimulation (TMS) is a non-invasive procedure where magnetic fields are used to stimulate nerve cells in the brain. Before beginning, you will sit comfortably in a chair, and a trained technician or doctor will place a coil on your head. This coil generates magnetic pulses that are targeted to specific areas of the brain linked to mood regulation, making it particularly useful for treating depression.

During the procedure, you might hear clicking sounds and feel a tapping sensation on your scalp. The intensity of the magnetic pulses can be adjusted based on your comfort level.

The procedure does not involve sedation, and you will remain awake and alert throughout. It is a relatively painless process, though some patients report mild discomfort or tingling at the site of stimulation.

Once the session is over, you can return to your regular activities immediately. TMS does not require any recovery time, making it convenient for those with busy schedules. The procedure is typically carried out on an outpatient basis, meaning you can go about your day as usual right after treatment.

The Initial Consultation And Assessment

Before starting TMS therapy, you'll need to have an initial consultation with a mental health professional. This meeting is essential to assess whether TMS is the right treatment for you, based on your medical history, current mental health status, and any previous treatments you've tried. The clinician will ask about your symptoms, any medications you are taking, and your overall mental health journey.

During this consultation, the doctor will also check if you have any contraindications to TMS, such as a history of seizures, metal implants in the head, or neurological disorders.

If you're deemed a good candidate for TMS, a treatment plan will be designed specifically for you. You will also discuss the risks, benefits, and potential side effects, ensuring you're fully informed before proceeding.

After the assessment, a physical exam or further tests may be conducted to measure the exact location in your brain that will receive stimulation. These preparatory steps are crucial for optimizing the effectiveness of the treatment and ensuring a safe and personalized experience.

Preparing For Your First TMS Session

In the days leading up to your first TMS session, there is not much you need to do in terms of preparation. You can eat, drink, and take your medications as usual. However, it is recommended to avoid consuming alcohol or using substances that might alter brain activity in the 24 hours before your appointment.

On the day of your session, wear comfortable clothing, and avoid any metal accessories like earrings, hairpins, or glasses, as the magnetic coil may interfere with these items.

You don't need to bring anything special with you to the appointment. Most importantly, try to arrive on time and relax, as the procedure is straightforward and non-invasive.

When you get to the clinic, the technician will help you settle into a comfortable chair, and the equipment will be adjusted to fit your head properly. You may feel a bit nervous if it's your first time, but the healthcare team will guide you through each step and answer any last-minute questions.

A Step-By-Step Guide To The Treatment Process

Once seated, the TMS technician will position the magnetic coil over your scalp.

The coil is typically placed near the prefrontal cortex, a brain area associated with mood regulation. The technician will adjust the device based on your head size and the specific target area that was determined during your initial assessment.

When the machine starts, it will send a series of magnetic pulses through the coil. Each pulse lasts only a few milliseconds, and you'll hear a clicking sound with each one. The session generally begins with a lower intensity, which may be increased as the treatment progresses to reach the optimal stimulation level.

During the session, which usually lasts about 20 to 40 minutes, you'll be sitting comfortably, and there's no need for you to do anything.

You can talk to the technician if you feel discomfort, though most people experience only mild sensations like tapping on the scalp. Once the treatment is finished, you'll be free to go about your day without any restrictions.

How Long Does Each Session Last?

TMS sessions typically last between 20 to 40 minutes, depending on the specific protocol being followed. The length of the session may vary slightly depending on the intensity of the stimulation and the area being targeted in your brain. For some patients, the sessions might start shorter and increase in length as their body adjusts to the treatment.

During the session, you will be sitting in a comfortable position while the machine does its work.

Although the clicking sounds and tapping sensations are repetitive, the process is generally well-tolerated by most patients.

If needed, the technician can adjust the settings to ensure that you remain comfortable throughout the session.

After the session, there's no need for recovery time, so you can leave immediately and continue with your daily activities. This makes TMS an appealing option for people with busy schedules, as it doesn't require downtime or lifestyle adjustments.

Frequency And Duration Of TMS Treatment Plans

A standard TMS treatment plan involves multiple sessions spread over several weeks. Typically, patients receive treatment five days a week for four to six weeks. The number of sessions required may vary based on individual needs and how well the patient responds to treatment. Some individuals may start noticing improvements after the first two weeks, while others might need the full course of treatment to feel significant changes.

Each treatment plan is tailored to the patient, with factors like the severity of symptoms and previous treatment history influencing the duration and frequency. After the initial treatment phase, some patients may require maintenance sessions, which are fewer in number but help sustain the benefits of the treatment.

Your doctor will continuously monitor your progress and may adjust the treatment schedule if necessary. TMS is considered a cumulative therapy, meaning that its effects build up over time, which is why it's crucial to adhere to the full treatment schedule for the best outcomes.

CHAPTER FIVE

TMS Machines And Equipment

Transcranial Magnetic Stimulation (TMS) machines are sophisticated devices used to non-invasively stimulate nerve cells in the brain, primarily to treat depression, anxiety, and other mental health conditions. The central component of any TMS system is the coil, which delivers magnetic pulses to specific brain regions.

These pulses are created by passing electric currents through the coil, generating magnetic fields that penetrate the skull and activate neural activity. Modern TMS machines are used in a clinical setting, often integrated with software that maps brain regions and tracks treatment progress.

TMS equipment comes with a variety of coil designs, each suited for different treatments and areas of the brain. The most commonly used coil is the figure-8 coil, known for its precision in targeting small areas of the brain. In addition to the coils, TMS machines also feature control units that regulate pulse frequency, duration, and intensity. Clinics may also use systems with neuronavigation technology, allowing clinicians to tailor treatments with pinpoint accuracy. These control systems ensure that patients receive the correct dosage of magnetic pulses according to their condition.

Safety is a crucial aspect of TMS machines, and modern devices are equipped with various safety features.

This includes emergency stop buttons, real-time monitoring of the magnetic field intensity, and built-in cooling systems to prevent overheating. While TMS is generally safe, the equipment is designed to minimize risks like discomfort or seizures. All TMS machines must be approved by regulatory bodies like the FDA to ensure they meet strict safety standards.

Overview Of TMS Devices Used In Clinics

Clinically, TMS devices are used primarily to treat major depressive disorder (MDD) and other neuropsychiatric conditions. These machines deliver high-frequency magnetic pulses to stimulate brain activity in regions such as the prefrontal cortex, which is often underactive in patients with depression.

Typically, treatment sessions last 20-40 minutes, and patients undergo several sessions per week for several weeks to achieve optimal results.

Each TMS session involves the patient sitting comfortably in a chair, where a clinician positions the magnetic coil over the patient's head. Advanced systems are designed to make this process seamless and comfortable, with some featuring built-in headrests to maintain proper coil positioning. During the procedure, patients may hear clicking sounds as the coil pulses and feel a tapping sensation on the scalp, but the process is generally pain-free.

There are several FDA-approved TMS devices, such as NeuroStar, BrainsWay, and

MagVenture. While they all operate on the same basic principle of magnetic pulse delivery, they differ in design, coil type, and flexibility in treatment protocols. For example, BrainsWay's Deep TMS system uses an H-coil that can stimulate deeper brain structures compared to standard figure-8 coils. This variety of devices gives clinicians the flexibility to choose the most appropriate system for their patient's specific needs.

Components Of A TMS Machine: Coils, Control Systems

The coil is the heart of a TMS machine and is responsible for generating the magnetic field that stimulates the brain. Coils come in various shapes and sizes, but the figure-8 coil is most common due to its ability to focus the magnetic field on smaller, more specific areas of the brain. The coil is placed on the patient's scalp during treatment, and electrical currents pass through it to create a magnetic field, which induces neural activity in targeted brain regions.

TMS control systems are equally important, as they regulate the machine's settings such as pulse intensity, frequency, and duration. These settings are adjusted based on the patient's treatment plan and condition.

Most TMS machines come with a user-friendly control panel or software interface that allows clinicians to easily modify treatment parameters in real-time. Some systems even have automated protocols based on the patient's diagnosis, ensuring consistent and accurate treatments.

Cooling systems are another vital component in many TMS machines. The continuous passage of electrical current can heat the coil, which may affect performance and patient comfort. Cooling mechanisms help maintain an optimal operating temperature, preventing overheating and ensuring the machine functions efficiently throughout the treatment session. Together, these components—coils, control systems, and cooling units—make TMS machines precise, safe, and reliable.

Safety Features Of Modern TMS Equipment

Modern TMS equipment is designed with patient safety as a top priority. One of the primary safety features is the inclusion of emergency stop buttons, allowing clinicians to immediately halt the treatment if the patient experiences discomfort or adverse reactions. This gives both patients and clinicians an added layer of control during sessions. Additionally, TMS machines monitor the magnetic field strength in real-time, ensuring that the pulses are delivered within safe and pre-programmed limits.

Another critical safety aspect is the prevention of overheating. As the coil generates pulses, heat can build up, potentially causing discomfort or malfunction.

To address this, TMS machines often include advanced cooling systems that regulate the coil's temperature, ensuring it remains safe for prolonged use. Furthermore, the machines are equipped with fail-safes, which automatically shut down the system if the equipment exceeds safe operating conditions.

Clinicians are also required to follow strict guidelines when administering TMS treatments, which include adjusting the magnetic pulse intensity to the patient's specific threshold. This ensures that the patient's brain receives the appropriate amount of stimulation without crossing into potentially harmful levels. Overall, the combination of built-in safety features and expert oversight makes modern TMS equipment safe for clinical use.

Innovations In TMS Technology

TMS technology is rapidly evolving, with innovations making treatments more effective and accessible. One of the key advancements is the development of deeper brain stimulation techniques. Traditional TMS machines stimulate superficial brain regions, but newer devices, like BrainsWay's Deep TMS, are designed to reach deeper neural structures, expanding the range of treatable conditions. This innovation allows for more comprehensive treatments, particularly for patients who do not respond to standard TMS.

Another significant innovation is neuronavigation, a technology that integrates real-time brain imaging with TMS to precisely target specific brain regions. This increases the accuracy of the treatments and improves patient outcomes, as clinicians can map and customize treatment to individual brain anatomy. By visualizing the exact location of brain regions, neuronavigation ensures the magnetic pulses are delivered to the correct area every time, which is especially useful for treating complex disorders.

Additionally, innovations in TMS have led to the creation of shorter treatment protocols, such as theta-burst stimulation, which can deliver the same therapeutic benefits in just a few minutes compared to the traditional 40-minute sessions. This makes the treatment process more convenient for patients while maintaining its effectiveness. As technology continues to advance, TMS is becoming a more versatile tool for treating a wide range of neurological and psychiatric disorders.

Home-Based TMS Devices: Are They Safe?

With advancements in technology, there has been increasing interest in home-based TMS devices, designed for self-administered treatment. These devices are typically less powerful than clinical TMS machines and are marketed as a convenient option for individuals suffering from mild depression or anxiety. However, their safety and effectiveness remain a topic of debate. Home-based TMS devices lack the real-time monitoring and precision controls found in clinical machines, which raise concerns about incorrect usage and potential side effects.

One of the key risks associated with home-based TMS devices is improper coil placement.

In a clinical setting, trained professionals carefully position the coil to ensure it targets the correct brain region. Without this expertise, users may unintentionally deliver the magnetic pulses to the wrong area, reducing the effectiveness of the treatment or causing adverse effects. Moreover, home devices do not usually have the advanced safety features of clinical machines, such as emergency stop buttons or automated monitoring systems.

While home-based TMS devices may offer convenience, they are not yet widely endorsed by medical professionals due to these safety concerns. Most clinicians recommend that TMS treatments be conducted in a clinical environment under the supervision of trained staff to ensure proper administration and safety. For those interested in home treatment, consulting with a healthcare provider is essential before starting any form of self-administered TMS therapy.

CHAPTER SIX

Benefits And Effectiveness Of TMS

Transcranial Magnetic Stimulation (TMS) is a non-invasive procedure that uses magnetic fields to stimulate nerve cells in the brain. It is primarily targeted at areas linked to mood regulation, like the prefrontal cortex, to improve mental health symptoms.

TMS is FDA-approved for treating depression, anxiety, and obsessive-compulsive disorder (OCD), and research is expanding its use to other conditions like chronic pain, PTSD, and addiction.

A key advantage of TMS is that it involves no surgery or anesthesia, unlike electroconvulsive therapy (ECT). The patient remains awake and alert during treatment, and each session typically takes 20-40 minutes. TMS is highly valued because it offers relief without the cognitive side effects often associated with medication, such as fatigue, memory issues, or emotional blunting.

Beyond mental health, TMS has also shown promise in neurorehabilitation, helping stroke survivors regain motor functions by stimulating areas of the brain related to movement.

Its effectiveness lies in its ability to enhance neuroplasticity—the brain's capacity to rewire itself. This makes TMS a powerful tool for both mental and neurological wellness.

Proven Benefits For Mental Health Conditions

TMS has become a lifeline for individuals with treatment-resistant depression (TRD) who don't respond to conventional medications or therapy. Studies show significant improvements in mood and functioning after several sessions, with patients reporting increased energy levels, better sleep, and reduced anxiety.

For those with anxiety disorders, TMS targets specific areas of the brain associated with overactivity and fear responses. In cases of OCD, it modulates circuits linked to compulsive behavior, gradually reducing intrusive thoughts and improving emotional regulation. Treatment plans are tailored to the patient's condition, ensuring targeted stimulation for the best outcomes.

TMS is also being explored for bipolar disorder, PTSD, and substance use disorders, offering a new horizon for patients with complex mental health needs. Unlike medications, which require long-term use, TMS provides a drug-free alternative with minimal side effects, making it a preferred option for people wary of chemical interventions.

Comparing TMS With Medications And Psychotherapy

Medications often come with side effects, including weight gain, sexual dysfunction, and emotional numbness, which can discourage patients from continuing treatment.

Psychotherapy requires ongoing engagement, and while effective, it may take months or years to yield significant results. TMS, on the other hand, offers a more direct and focused approach to brain modulation.

In many cases, TMS is used as an adjunct to existing therapies, complementing medication or psychotherapy. For example, patients who have plateaued in therapy might undergo TMS to stimulate brain function and re-engage with their emotional processing. This synergy often accelerates recovery and boosts overall treatment outcomes.

The non-invasive nature of TMS makes it an attractive option for individuals looking for quick symptom relief without the risk of addiction or tolerance seen with some medications. TMS offers a practical bridge between pharmacological treatment and talk therapy, especially for those with long-standing mental health conditions.

Success Rates And Patient Experiences

Clinical studies suggest that up to 70% of patients with treatment-resistant depression experience significant symptom improvement after TMS therapy, with around 50% achieving complete remission. Patients often describe the process as pain-free, feeling only a light tapping sensation on the scalp during the procedure.

Success stories emphasize the emotional and physical transformations many individuals experience after several weeks of TMS.

Improvements in motivation, cognitive clarity, and social engagement are common, making it easier for patients to return to work and daily activities. For those suffering from anxiety, many report feeling calmer and better equipped to manage stress.

However, TMS is not a universal solution, and outcomes can vary. Some patients may require booster sessions to maintain their progress, while others might need to combine TMS with medications or therapy. Overall, the patient feedback on TMS is overwhelmingly positive, particularly for those who had previously exhausted other treatment options.

How Soon Will You See The Results?
TMS is not an instant solution, and the timeline for results varies between individuals.

Many patients begin to notice subtle improvements, such as better sleep or increased concentration, after the first week of treatment. However, meaningful changes in mood and mental health typically occur after 4-6 weeks of regular sessions.

A standard TMS course involves 5 sessions per week, lasting 4 to 6 weeks, though some providers offer accelerated protocols. Patients are advised to track their symptoms throughout the process, as the shifts in mood can be gradual. Progress can often feel subtle at first but tends to build over time, leading to noticeable improvements by the end of the treatment cycle.

For some individuals, booster sessions may be recommended months after the initial course to sustain the positive effects. While TMS offers long-term benefits, regular check-ins with a mental health provider ensure that progress continues and that any emerging symptoms are addressed promptly.

Maintaining Mental Health After TMS

Post-TMS care is essential to maintaining the benefits of the treatment. Patients are encouraged to continue engaging in healthy practices, such as regular exercise, balanced nutrition, and sufficient sleep, which support overall mental well-being.

Additionally, incorporating relaxation techniques, like mindfulness or yoga, helps reduce stress and enhances emotional stability.

For those already undergoing therapy, it's beneficial to continue attending sessions after TMS. Therapy provides a space to process changes in mood and behavior and to reinforce new coping strategies.

Some patients might also maintain low-dose medication to prevent symptom recurrence, though many find they can reduce or discontinue medication over time.

Regular follow-ups with the treatment provider allow for personalized care, and in some cases, patients might return for booster sessions if symptoms reappear. TMS is most effective when combined with a proactive approach to mental health, ensuring the long-lasting benefits of the treatment are preserved.

CHAPTER SEVEN

Common Concerns And Side Effects

Many individuals have concerns about the safety and potential side effects of Transcranial Magnetic Stimulation (TMS), especially when considering it for the first time. TMS is a non-invasive procedure that uses magnetic fields to stimulate nerve cells in the brain. It is primarily used to treat conditions like depression, anxiety, and OCD. While generally considered safe, like any medical treatment, TMS has potential side effects that patients should be aware of.

The most common side effects are mild and typically occur during or immediately after treatment. These can include scalp discomfort or a tingling sensation at the treatment site, headaches, and slight dizziness. The intensity of these side effects usually decreases as the brain adjusts to the stimulation over the course of several sessions. Most side effects are manageable and tend to resolve quickly after the treatment session ends.

While serious side effects are rare, it's important to communicate with the healthcare provider throughout the treatment process. Monitoring any unusual symptoms, especially if they persist, is critical. Side effects should be reported so adjustments can be made, such as reducing the intensity of the magnetic pulses.

Is TMS Painful Or Uncomfortable?
TMS is generally not painful, but some people may experience mild discomfort during the procedure.

The magnetic pulses delivered to the brain through the scalp can create a tapping or tingling sensation. This sensation is usually described as tolerable but may be slightly uncomfortable for some. The discomfort tends to be most noticeable during the first few sessions and diminishes as the patient gets used to the procedure.

The device used in TMS has a coil that is placed on the scalp near the forehead. When the machine is activated, patients may hear clicking sounds, similar to an MRI machine, and feel a rhythmic tapping at the treatment site. This sensation can vary in intensity depending on the individual's sensitivity and the location being stimulated.

Sessions last about 20-40 minutes, and breaks can be taken if needed.

To minimize discomfort, healthcare providers can adjust the strength of the magnetic pulses or offer breaks during treatment. Pain relievers, like over-the-counter headache medication, can also be taken beforehand if recommended by the doctor. Most patients find the discomfort to be manageable and not a reason to discontinue treatment.

Potential Side Effects: What You Should Know

Though TMS is considered a safe treatment, it's essential to understand its potential side effects. The most common side effect is mild headache, which usually subsides shortly after treatment.

Some people may also experience muscle twitching or discomfort at the site where the magnet is applied, but this is generally short-lived.

Rare but more severe side effects include seizures, which occur in less than 0.1% of patients, particularly those with a history of epilepsy or other neurological conditions. Additionally, some individuals may experience mood swings, especially if they have a history of bipolar disorder. It is important for individuals undergoing TMS to communicate any changes in mood or behavior to their doctor, as these can be managed effectively with adjustments to the treatment plan.

In very rare cases, patients may report worsening depression symptoms during the early stages of treatment. However, these usually improve as the therapy continues. The side effects of TMS are typically mild compared to other treatments like medication, making it a favorable option for individuals who have not responded well to antidepressants.

Managing Minor Side Effects Like Headaches

Headaches are the most common minor side effect associated with TMS therapy. They typically occur due to the stimulation of muscles and nerves in the scalp during the procedure.

For most patients, the headaches are mild and temporary, fading within a few hours of the session. However, in some cases, they can be more persistent and uncomfortable, especially during the initial treatments.

To manage headaches, patients are often advised to take over-the-counter pain relievers, such as ibuprofen or acetaminophen, before or after their sessions. Drinking plenty of water and maintaining a relaxed posture during the treatment may also help alleviate the discomfort. Some clinics may offer adjustments to the magnetic pulse strength to reduce the likelihood of headaches, especially if a patient is particularly sensitive to the stimulation.

If headaches persist or worsen, it's important to inform the healthcare provider. Adjusting the intensity of the magnetic pulses or the frequency of the sessions can make a significant difference. In most cases, as patients progress through their treatment plan, the headaches become less frequent and less severe.

Who Should Avoid TMS? Contraindications

While TMS is considered safe for many people, there are certain conditions and medical histories that may make someone ineligible for the treatment. The presence of metal in or near the head is one of the most significant contraindications.

For example, individuals with metal implants in the brain, cochlear implants, or aneurysm clips should not undergo TMS. The magnetic pulses could interfere with these devices or pose a risk of injury.

Additionally, people with a history of seizures or epilepsy should consult closely with their doctor before considering TMS, as there is a small risk of seizure during the procedure. TMS may also be inappropriate for individuals with other neurological conditions or brain injuries that could be aggravated by the stimulation. Pregnant women should also discuss TMS with their healthcare provider, as the safety of TMS during pregnancy has not been thoroughly studied.

Other factors that may exclude someone from receiving TMS include severe anxiety or agitation that makes it difficult to remain still during the sessions. Patients need to undergo a thorough screening process to determine whether TMS is safe and suitable for their condition. If any contraindications exist, alternative treatments should be explored.

Can TMS Cause Memory Loss Or Brain Damage?

One common misconception about TMS is that it can cause memory loss or brain damage. In reality, there is no evidence to suggest that TMS negatively affects memory or causes any form of brain injury. Unlike electroconvulsive therapy (ECT), which can impact memory, TMS uses magnetic pulses that are more targeted and less invasive, meaning it does not carry the same risks.

Some studies suggest that TMS may even improve cognitive function, especially in areas related to attention and memory, as part of its positive effects on depression and other conditions. Memory issues are generally not reported as a side effect of TMS. However, individuals need to track any cognitive changes they notice and discuss them with their healthcare provider to ensure the treatment is working as intended.

Overall, TMS is considered a safe option for most patients, and concerns about brain damage are unfounded. The magnetic pulses used in TMS are designed to stimulate specific areas of the brain without causing harm, making it a non-invasive and safe treatment option for various mental health conditions.

CHAPTER EIGHT

Cost, Insurance, And Accessibility

How Much Does TMS Treatment Cost?

The cost of Transcranial Magnetic Stimulation (TMS) can vary depending on the clinic, region, and specific treatment plan. On average, a full course of TMS therapy, which typically includes 20-30 sessions over several weeks, ranges from $6,000 to $12,000.

Each session might cost between $300 and $500, depending on factors like the equipment used and the provider's experience. While this may seem expensive, many people find the long-term benefits outweigh the initial investment, especially for those who haven't responded to medication.

TMS pricing is also influenced by the type of TMS machine used, as some machines offer more advanced targeting or comfort features. It is also possible to see variability in cost based on whether the treatment is being used for conditions beyond depression, such as OCD or PTSD, which may require more specialized approaches. Clinics often provide estimates during initial consultations to ensure clarity on pricing.

Before beginning treatment, it is important to ask about any additional costs, such as follow-up sessions or potential additional therapies. Some clinics may offer discounts for upfront payment, but it's essential to ask what is included in the quoted price and whether additional services like consultation fees or administrative costs will be charged separately.

Insurance Coverage For TMS: What's Included?

Insurance coverage for TMS therapy depends on the specific insurance provider and plan. Many major insurers, such as Blue Cross Blue Shield, Aetna, and UnitedHealthcare, cover TMS therapy for treatment-resistant depression when standard treatments like medication and psychotherapy have failed. However, the patient usually needs to meet certain criteria, including a history of trying multiple antidepressants without success, and sometimes documentation of failed psychotherapy. Some plans may cover part of the treatment, leaving the patient responsible for a copay or coinsurance fee for each session. It is important to confirm whether your insurance covers the full course of treatment or only a specific number of sessions. Coverage for conditions other than depression, like anxiety or OCD, may not always be included without prior approval or additional evidence of medical necessity.

To make sure you maximize your insurance benefits, always check with your provider before starting TMS therapy. Many TMS clinics will also assist in navigating insurance pre-authorization and handling the necessary paperwork to confirm coverage. Some clinics have dedicated staff to help patients communicate with their insurance companies about coverage.

Finding TMS Clinics And Providers Near You

Finding a TMS clinic nearby is usually the first step after deciding to pursue treatment. Many mental health professionals, including psychiatrists, offer TMS therapy in their practice or can refer you to specialized TMS clinics. It's important to choose a provider who is experienced and certified in administering TMS, as the procedure requires technical precision and individualized care.

Online directories, like those provided by the Clinical TMS Society or the American Psychiatric Association, can help in locating certified providers. A simple internet search using terms like "TMS clinics near me" can also yield local results.

You can also ask your general practitioner or therapist for recommendations based on your specific needs and diagnosis.

When choosing a clinic, consider factors such as proximity to your home or workplace, the experience of the staff, and the availability of flexible scheduling options. It's also essential to ask whether the clinic offers the specific TMS protocol that best suits your condition, as there are different types of TMS available, like deep TMS or repetitive TMS (rTMS).

Financial Assistance And Payment Plans
For those concerned about the high upfront costs of TMS therapy, many clinics offer financial assistance or flexible payment plans.

These plans typically allow patients to spread the cost of treatment over several months rather than paying the entire amount upfront. Clinics may partner with third-party financing companies that specialize in healthcare loans, offering low-interest rates for qualified individuals.

Additionally, some clinics provide sliding scale fees based on income or offer discounts for individuals without insurance coverage. It's always helpful to ask the clinic if they have any special pricing options or payment plans before starting treatment. If you are struggling financially, explaining your situation may help open up additional options for making treatment more affordable.

Nonprofit organizations and mental health charities occasionally offer grants or funding for TMS treatment, especially for individuals facing financial hardship. Some patient advocacy groups also help connect individuals to resources that might lower the cost of TMS treatment, making it more accessible to those who need it most.

Does Medicare Or Medicaid Cover TMS?

Yes, Medicare covers TMS therapy for treatment-resistant depression, though the process may require certain prerequisites.

Medicare typically mandates that patients try multiple antidepressant medications and psychotherapy before approving TMS treatment.

In most cases, Medicare covers 80% of the cost of TMS once it's deemed medically necessary, with patients responsible for the remaining 20%, which can be offset by supplemental insurance.

Medicaid coverage for TMS, however, varies significantly depending on the state. In some states, Medicaid may cover TMS therapy for treatment-resistant depression, but the approval process can be more challenging, with stricter guidelines and more paperwork. It's best to consult with a Medicaid case manager or your local Medicaid office to understand the exact requirements and potential for coverage.

To ensure coverage through Medicare or Medicaid, it's important to work closely with your healthcare provider, who can document your medical history and submit the necessary paperwork for pre-authorization. Many TMS clinics are experienced in handling Medicare and Medicaid claims and can assist with navigating the system to ensure timely and appropriate care.

CHAPTER NINE

FAQs: Frequently Asked Questions About TMS

Transcranial Magnetic Stimulation (TMS) is a non-invasive treatment that uses magnetic fields to stimulate nerve cells in the brain. One of the most common questions is how long treatment takes. A typical session lasts around 20-40 minutes, with most patients undergoing daily sessions over a period of 4 to 6 weeks. Another question people ask is if TMS is painful. The answer is no, but patients may feel tapping or twitching sensations on the scalp during the process.

People also ask about side effects. The side effects of TMS are generally mild, including scalp discomfort, headaches, or slight lightheadedness, and they often fade after the session. There's a concern about whether TMS is safe for everyone. While TMS is safe, it's not recommended for people with certain types of metal implants, pacemakers, or seizure disorders.

Lastly, many wonder if TMS is covered by insurance. In many cases, it is, especially for patients with treatment-resistant depression, but it's essential to confirm coverage with your provider beforehand. Consulting a TMS provider is the best way to address specific questions and concerns.

What Does TMS Feel Like During Treatment?

During TMS treatment, you'll be seated comfortably in a chair while a coil is placed on your scalp, typically targeting areas linked to depression. As the machine starts, you'll hear a clicking sound and feel a tapping sensation on your head, which can feel like gentle, repetitive taps. The sensation can be odd at first but generally becomes tolerable after a few moments. Some people liken it to the feeling of a light knock or a firm tapping on the head.

The intensity of the stimulation can be adjusted to make you more comfortable. If the tapping feels too intense, you can ask the technician to make adjustments. In addition to the tapping, some patients experience muscle twitches in their faces, but this is completely normal and will stop once the session is over.

Most people do not feel any pain during TMS, though mild scalp discomfort is common at first. As the sessions continue, the sensation usually becomes more familiar, and most patients find it easy to relax during the treatment.

How Do I Know If I'm A Good Candidate?

TMS is primarily used for individuals with major depressive disorder who have not responded well to medications or therapy. To determine if you're a good candidate, your doctor will assess your medical history, including any previous treatments for depression. If you've tried at least two antidepressants without significant improvement, TMS may be a suitable option.

It's also a good choice for patients looking for a non-invasive treatment option.

However, TMS isn't recommended for everyone. If you have a history of seizures, certain types of brain injuries, or metal implants near the head (such as aneurysm clips or cochlear implants), you may not be eligible. People with pacemakers or other implanted devices might also be excluded due to the magnetic nature of the treatment.

A consultation with a TMS provider will help you understand if this treatment is appropriate for your condition. They will conduct a thorough evaluation to ensure the treatment is safe and effective for your specific case.

Can I Combine TMS With Medications?

Yes, TMS can be combined with medications. Many patients continue taking their prescribed antidepressants during their TMS treatment. Since TMS works differently from medications—by stimulating targeted areas of the brain with magnetic pulses—it can complement the effects of drugs. Often, patients find that the combination leads to better results, especially when previous medication treatments alone have not worked.

Before starting TMS, it's important to inform your healthcare provider about all medications you're currently taking. Certain drugs, such as seizure medications, might require adjustments before beginning treatment. Your doctor will guide you on the best course of action based on your medication regimen and medical history.

Some patients find that after successful TMS treatments, they can reduce or even stop taking their antidepressant medications. However, any changes to your medication should only be done under the supervision of your healthcare provider.

Will I Need Maintenance Tms After Treatment?

After completing the initial TMS treatment, some patients may require maintenance sessions to prevent symptoms from returning. Maintenance TMS is typically offered on a less frequent basis, such as weekly or monthly sessions, depending on your response to the initial treatment. Your doctor will monitor your progress and determine if and when maintenance treatments are needed.

For many patients, the effects of TMS can last several months or even longer after the initial treatment course. However, because depression can be a chronic condition, some individuals benefit from periodic "booster" sessions to maintain their mental health. These sessions are usually shorter and less frequent than the original treatment series.

Discussing your long-term mental health goals with your provider will help you understand if maintenance TMS is necessary for you. They will create a personalized plan to ensure sustained improvement and monitor your progress closely.

Is There Any Downtime After TMS Sessions?

One of the benefits of TMS is that there's no downtime after sessions. You can return to your normal activities immediately after each treatment. Patients often drive themselves to and from the sessions without any issues. There are no lingering effects like sedation or memory problems, making it easy to incorporate TMS into your daily routine.

While some patients experience mild headaches or scalp discomfort after treatment, these side effects typically resolve quickly and don't interfere with daily activities. If discomfort occurs, over-the-counter pain relievers can usually manage any minor aches.

Because TMS doesn't involve anesthesia or any invasive procedures, it's a convenient option for those looking for an effective depression treatment without the need to take time off work or other responsibilities.

CHAPTER TEN

Future Trends And Innovations In TMS

Transcranial Magnetic Stimulation (TMS) continues to evolve, with promising trends emerging. One area of development is the use of more precise, focused magnetic pulses. This allows for targeted stimulation of specific brain regions with better accuracy, reducing side effects while improving effectiveness. Portable and wearable TMS devices are also being explored, allowing patients to potentially receive treatments in non-clinical settings, such as at home, providing more flexibility and convenience.

Another innovation is the expansion of TMS into different treatment areas beyond depression. Researchers are exploring TMS for conditions like chronic pain, migraines, anxiety, PTSD, and even neurodegenerative disorders like Parkinson's disease. By fine-tuning protocols, the future of TMS could involve a much broader range of applications, helping more individuals with diverse mental health and neurological conditions.

As technology advances, integrating TMS with real-time brain imaging could enhance outcomes. By monitoring the brain's response to stimulation in real-time, clinicians can adjust the treatment on the spot, ensuring more precise, effective sessions. These innovations make TMS a continuously evolving therapy that holds great potential for the future.

Research Into New Applications For TMS

Recent research is pushing the boundaries of what TMS can treat. While TMS is FDA-approved for major depressive disorder, studies are investigating its effectiveness in treating other psychiatric and neurological conditions. Early trials suggest promising outcomes for anxiety disorders, PTSD, addiction, and even obsessive-compulsive disorder (OCD). This expanding research highlights TMS as a versatile tool with the potential to revolutionize treatments across many mental health areas.

In the neurological domain, TMS is being tested for conditions like Alzheimer's disease, stroke recovery, and chronic pain management.

For example, TMS may help stimulate brain areas involved in motor control, aiding recovery for stroke patients. Similarly, research is underway to see how TMS can reduce pain signals in chronic pain sufferers, offering a non-invasive alternative to medications.

These new applications are in the experimental phase, but early results are promising. As clinical trials progress, more conditions may receive approval for TMS, broadening its scope and providing non-drug alternatives for conditions that are traditionally difficult to treat.

Personalized TMS: Tailoring Treatment To Individuals

Personalized TMS is an emerging approach that tailors treatment to each individual's unique brain activity and condition. Instead of using a one-size-fits-all protocol, personalized TMS analyzes a patient's specific brain patterns through imaging techniques like MRI. This allows clinicians to adjust the intensity, frequency, and placement of the magnetic pulses based on the patient's needs, resulting in more targeted and effective therapy.

By customizing treatment parameters, personalized TMS can optimize outcomes, especially for patients who might not respond well to traditional TMS settings. For instance, someone with severe depression might benefit from higher-frequency stimulation, while another patient with anxiety could require a gentler approach. Personalization ensures that each patient receives the most effective, comfortable treatment possible.

Advances in neuroimaging and data collection are driving this shift toward personalization. As the field progresses, more tools will likely emerge to allow even greater customization, offering hope to patients whose conditions have proven resistant to standard therapies.

Combining TMS With Other Therapies (CBT, EMDR)

TMS is increasingly being combined with other therapeutic modalities, such as Cognitive Behavioral Therapy (CBT) and Eye Movement Desensitization and Reprocessing (EMDR). The idea is to amplify the benefits of both treatments by addressing neurological and psychological aspects simultaneously.

For instance, while TMS stimulates brain areas involved in mood regulation, CBT can help patients develop healthier thought patterns, complementing the brain stimulation.

In the case of PTSD or trauma, combining TMS with EMDR can provide a dual approach to recovery. TMS may help reduce the physiological symptoms associated with trauma, like hypervigilance, while EMDR helps reprocess traumatic memories. This integrated approach can make the therapy more effective, especially for patients with complex mental health conditions.

Practically, a patient might receive TMS sessions several times a week while also engaging in psychotherapy. This combination targets both the brain's neurochemistry and the cognitive patterns underlying their symptoms, offering a comprehensive treatment plan that addresses multiple facets of mental health recovery.

The Role Of AI And Data In Improving TMS Outcomes

Artificial intelligence (AI) and data analytics are becoming vital tools in enhancing TMS outcomes. AI can help by analyzing vast amounts of patient data to identify patterns that human clinicians might miss.

This data-driven approach allows for more precise adjustments to TMS protocols based on a patient's unique brain activity, increasing the likelihood of success and reducing trial-and-error in treatment.

AI can also predict which patients are more likely to respond well to TMS, using machine learning algorithms to process past treatment data. This enables clinicians to make more informed decisions, selecting the most effective treatment parameters from the start. In this way, AI helps personalize treatments on a deeper level, improving overall success rates.

Additionally, data collection during TMS sessions can be used to refine protocols continuously. By monitoring patient responses in real-time and feeding this data into AI systems, TMS treatments can evolve dynamically, improving both safety and efficacy over time.

Future Accessibility: Lowering Costs And Increasing Reach

One of the biggest challenges with TMS today is its cost and accessibility. However, as technology advances and more clinics adopt TMS, the cost is expected to decrease. Innovations, such as portable and at-home TMS devices, are being developed, which could significantly reduce the need for clinic-based treatments and lower the overall financial burden on patients.

Another way accessibility could improve is through insurance coverage. As more conditions become FDA-approved for TMS treatment, insurance providers may be more likely to cover these therapies, making them more affordable for a larger group of people.

Lowering the barriers to access can make TMS a mainstream treatment option for various mental health and neurological conditions.

Telemedicine platforms are also making it easier to access TMS consultations, with remote sessions potentially becoming more viable as the technology improves. The goal is to make TMS not only more affordable but also more widely available to underserved populations, bridging the gap in mental health treatment access across regions and income levels.

Conclusion

Transcranial Magnetic Stimulation (TMS) is a non-invasive procedure that uses magnetic fields to stimulate nerve cells in the brain, primarily for the treatment of neurological and psychiatric conditions such as depression, anxiety, and chronic pain. By the end of this comprehensive guide, it is clear that TMS has emerged as a revolutionary technique with promising results, especially in patients who do not respond to traditional treatments like medication or psychotherapy.

This guide highlights the efficacy and safety of TMS, showing that it offers a non-pharmacological option with minimal side effects compared to more invasive treatments like electroconvulsive therapy (ECT). For many, TMS has proven to be a life-changing therapy, providing relief from symptoms of treatment-resistant depression and other mood disorders. The mechanism of action involves stimulating specific regions of the brain, such as the prefrontal cortex, to restore normal neural activity.

However, this guide also stresses that TMS is not a one-size-fits-all solution. Results can vary depending on individual brain chemistry, the specific condition being treated, and the frequency or intensity of the sessions. While the long-term effects and potential uses of TMS continue to be explored, patients need to consult with medical professionals to determine if it is the right option for their specific needs.

In conclusion, TMS represents a significant advancement in the field of neurostimulation, offering hope to individuals who have not found success with other treatments. Its ongoing development suggests that it could become an even more widely adopted treatment method in the future, potentially expanding beyond psychiatric conditions to other neurological disorders as research progresses.

THE END

www.ingramcontent.com/pod-product-compliance
Lightning Source LLC
Chambersburg PA
CBHW052323220526
45472CB00001B/240

* 9 7 9 8 3 0 0 7 7 5 2 9 2 *